YOUR KNOWLEDGE HAS VALUE

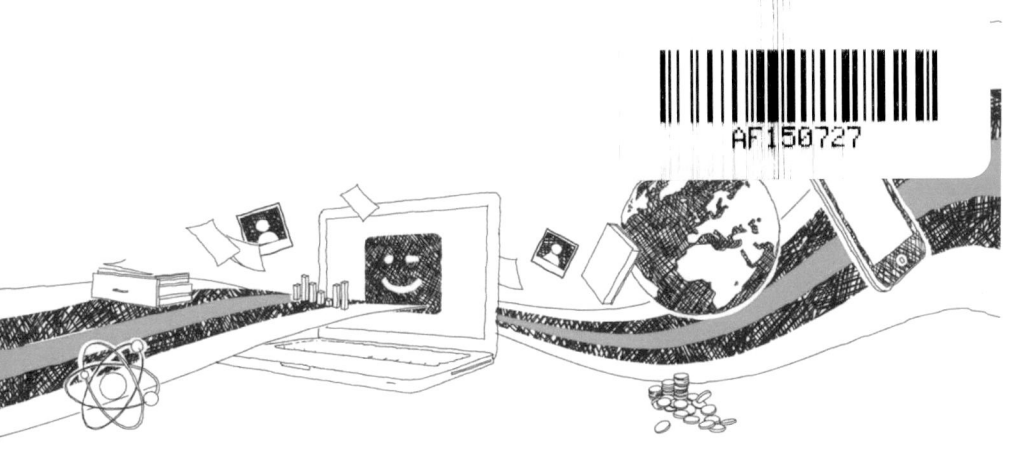
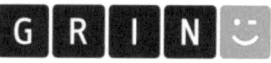

Bibliographic information published by the German National Library:

The German National Library lists this publication in the National Bibliography; detailed bibliographic data are available on the Internet at http://dnb.dnb.de .

Imprint:

Copyright © 2017 GRIN Verlag
Print and binding: Books on Demand GmbH, Norderstedt Germany
ISBN: 9783668575899

This book at GRIN:

https://www.grin.com/document/381285

Patrick Kimuyu

Burkitt Lymphoma. Forms, Effects, Risk Factors, Treatment

GRIN Verlag

GRIN - Your knowledge has value

Since its foundation in 1998, GRIN has specialized in publishing academic texts by students, college teachers and other academics as e-book and printed book. The website www.grin.com is an ideal platform for presenting term papers, final papers, scientific essays, dissertations and specialist books.

Visit us on the internet:

http://www.grin.com/

http://www.facebook.com/grincom

http://www.twitter.com/grin_com

Burkitt Lymphoma

Name: Patrick K. Kimuyu

Summary 2

Introduction 4

Forms of Burkitt Lymphoma and their Effects on Body Physiology 4

Anatomical Regions Affected by Burkitt Lymphoma 6

Risk Factors of Burkitt Lymphoma 7

Pathophysiology 8

Physiological Effects of Burkitt Lymphoma Symptoms 10

Treatment of Burkitt Lymphoma: How Therapies Affect Physiology 11

Conclusion 12

References 13

Summary

Burkitt lymphoma has become one of the most prevalent cancers in the last three decades in which the number of people with the disease has increased, especially in Africa. Research indicates that, burkitt lymphoma has emerged to be the fastest growing tumor among humans. Burkitt lymphoma was identified in 1956 by Denis Burkitt, and it is one of the principal forms on non-Hodgkin's lymphoma, which affect immune cells. Lymphocytes, primarily the B-cells of the immune system which are involved in cell-mediated immune response during pathogenic infections are affected. In most cases, the prevalence of the disease is enhanced by infections which weaken the immune system. For instance, malaria, Epstein-Barr viral infection and HIV are some of the diseases associated with a decrease of the immune system response. However, the physiology and anatomy of Burkitt lymphoma encompasses diverse aspects compared to other forms cancer.

The epidemiology and geographical distribution of Burkitt lymphoma depend on the form of the disease involved. Currently, three principal forms of the disease have been identified, and their prevalence and incidence trends manifest diverse variations, especially with regard to the population affected and the principal causes.

There are three forms of Burkitt lymphoma: sporadic Burkitt lymphoma, endemic Burkitt lymphoma and immunodeficiency-related Burkitt lymphoma.

Sporadic Burkitt lymphoma has been found to have a global distribution in which it accounts for about 2% of all lymphoma cases among adults. In some developed countries such as UK and the U.S, sporadic Burkitt lymphoma is relatively prevalent in children in which 40% of lymphoma cases occur in children.

Endemic Burkitt lymphoma is usually found, predominantly in equatorial Africa where it affects children more than adults. It is worth noting that, endemic Burkitt lymphoma exhibits diverse prevalence trends in regard to gender in which it is more prevalent in African boys than girls, especially within the age of 4-7 years.

Immunodeficiency-related Burkitt lymphoma occurs in people with suppressed immunity, and it does not exhibit demographic and geographical restrictions. Ordinarily, this variant of lymphoma occurs in patients with HIV/AIDS and organ-transplant patients.

From an anatomical perspective, Burkitt lymphoma affects body organs, which have the lymphoid tissue. The lymphoid tissue comprises of immune stem cells, primarily the T lymphocytes (T cells) and B lymphocytes (B cells). Some of the organs affected by Burkitt lymphoma are made up of the lymphoid tissue.

Currently, an array of risk factors for Burkitt lymphoma has been identified although the mechanisms behind some risk factors remain unknown. Burkitt lymphoma exhibit similar features to those observed in other forms of cancer although they differ significantly in regard to etiology and risk factors. Some of the risk factors which are believed to increase an individual's chance of developing Burkitt lymphoma include age, gender, immune system deficiency, infections and exposure to certain chemicals.

For purposes of pathophysiology, it is believed that oncogenes and suppressor genes play a significant role in DNA changes observed in Burkitt lymphoma. In theory, oncogenes are responsible for speeding up cell division for cellular proliferation or organ development. On the other hand, suppressor genes, also known as tumor suppressor genes are responsible for controlling cell death by slowing down cell division. These two processes occur uniformly to ensure efficient growth and development, but fatal consequences occur when imbalances are experienced.

Introduction

Burkitt lymphoma has become one of the most prevalent cancers in the past two decades in which the number of people with the disease has increased, especially in Africa. Research indicates that, burkitt lymphoma has emerged to be the fastest growing tumor among humans. Burkitt lymphoma was identified in 1956 by Denis Burkitt, and it is one of the principal forms on non-Hodgkin's lymphoma, which affect immune cells. Epidemiological reports indicate that, Burkitt lymphoma is more prevalent in malaria endemic regions than other regions although it greatest impact is experienced in Africa where it affects children who are also experiencing episodes of malaria and Epstein-Barr viral infection. Epstein-Barr virus is believed to be the principal cause of infectious mononucleosis, which leads to the transformation of B-cells into tumor cells, especially following malaria episode which weakens the immune system. This is probably the reason as to why 98% of Burkitt lymphoma cases in Africa are linked to Epstein-Barr infection. Elsewhere in the U.S, the incidence of Burkitt lymphoma accounts for about 1,200 people annually in which 59% of all the patients diagnosed with the disease being adults above the age of 40 years (WebMD, 2013).

In Burkitt lymphoma, lymphocytes, primarily the B-cells of the immune system which are involved in cell-mediated immune response during pathogenic infections are affected. In most cases, the prevalence of the disease is enhanced by infections which weaken the immune system. For instance, malaria, Epstein-Barr viral infection and HIV are some of the diseases associated with a decrease of the immune system response. In addition, therapies which are immune-suppressive, especially those involved in organ transplantation to prevent transplant rejection and highly-active antiretroviral therapy (HAART) used for HIV/AIDS treatment facilitate the formation of cancerous B-cells. However, the physiology and anatomy of Burkitt lymphoma encompasses diverse aspects compared to other forms cancer. Therefore, this research paper will provide an overview on Burkitt lymphoma disease and its pathophysiology.

Forms of Burkitt Lymphoma and their Effects on Body Physiology

It has been found out that the epidemiology and geographical distribution of Burkitt lymphoma depend on the form of the disease involved. Currently, three principal forms of the disease have been identified, and their prevalence and incidence trends manifest diverse variations, especially with regard to the population affected and the principal causes.

World Health Organization has categorized the principal forms of Burkitt lymphoma as sporadic Burkitt lymphoma, endemic Burkitt lymphoma and immunodeficiency-related Burkitt lymphoma. Sporadic Burkitt lymphoma has been found to have a global distribution in which it accounts for about 2% of all lymphoma cases among adults (American Cancer Society, 2013). In some developed countries such as UK and the U.S, sporadic Burkitt lymphoma is relatively prevalent in children in which 40% of lymphoma cases occur in children (WebMD, 2013). This form of Burkitt lymphoma is associated with EBV (Epstein - Barr virus) infection although there are other unknown etiological causes. In regard to the body anatomy, sporadic Burkitt lymphoma has been found to affect the lower abdomen. In most cases, it occurs in lymph nodes, which innervate the junction between large intestines and small intestines (Lights & Yu, 2012).

Endemic Burkitt lymphoma is usually found, predominantly in equatorial Africa where it affects children more than adults. It is worth noting that, endemic Burkitt lymphoma exhibits diverse prevalence trends in regard to gender in which it is more prevalent in African boys than girls, especially within the age of 4-7 years (WebMD, 2013). It affects jaw and facial bone although it may involve breasts, kidneys, ovaries and the small intestine (Lights & Yu, 2012).

On the other hand, immunodeficiency-related Burkitt lymphoma occurs in people with suppressed immunity and it does not exhibit demographic and geographical restrictions. Ordinarily, this variant of lymphoma occurs in patients with HIV/AIDS and organ-transplant patients. It is estimated that, immunodeficiency-related Burkitt lymphoma accounts for about 40% of all non-Hodgkin lymphoma cases reported in HIV/AIDS patients (Jaffe, 2001). It is also believed to occur in patients with immunodeficiency-related congenital conditions. In theory, immunodeficiency-related Burkitt lymphoma occurs in HIV/AIDS and organ-transplant patients because they are exposed to immune-suppressive drugs. In HIV/AIDS patients, HAART drugs weaken the immune system leading to the proliferation of invasive cancerous B-cells (Lights & Yu, 2012). On the other hand, immune-suppressive drugs administered to organ-transplant patients impair immune stem responses to Epstein-Barr virus, which acts as the principal etiological agent in Burkitt lymphoma disease. In practice, organ transplant is associated to the immune system response in which the body accepts or rejects the transplant. Therefore, immunosuppressive drugs are used to prevent the patient's body from rejecting the transplant after recognizing it as 'foreign'.

Anatomical Regions Affected by Burkitt Lymphoma

In general, Burkitt lymphoma affects body organs, which have the lymphoid tissue. The lymphoid tissue comprises of immune stem cells, primarily the T lymphocytes (T cells) and B lymphocytes (B cells). Ordinarily, Burkitt lymphoma involves B cells exclusively; thus, it affects that manner in which the immune system responds to viral and bacterial infections through the production of antibodies (American Cancer Society, 2013).

Some of the organs affected by Burkitt lymphoma are made up of the lymphoid tissue. This is the principal reason as to why lymphomas can be found in virtually all parts of the body because they contain the lymphoid tissue. However, it occurs mostly in lymph nodes, spleen, digestive tract, bone marrow and adenoids.

Lymph nodes are concentrated in the chest, pelvis and the abdomen and they are involved in fighting infections. It is believed that, Epstein-Barr infection causes the lymph nodes to enlarge, a condition referred to as hyperplastic which advances into tumor cells, especially when untreated (American Cancer Society, 2013). Therefore, the enlargement of lymph nodes serves as the principal approach for the detection of Burkitt lymphoma, as well as other non-Hodgkin's lymphomas.

Spleen and the thymus serve as secondary lymphoid organs in which B cells and T cells undergo differentiation for use in the immune system responses. As such, they play pivotal roles in enhancing the functioning of the immune system, although the thymus gland is not involved in Burkitt lymphoma. On the other hand, adenoids and tonsils help in producing antibodies which are used in fighting infections as it is the case for Epstein-Barr viral infection which causes enlargement of these lymphoid organs owing to the growth of tumors associated to B cells. This is the reason as to why endemic Burkitt lymphoma affects the neck region where adenoids and tonsils are located.

Lymphoid tissue is also found in the bone marrow and the entire gastrointestinal tract where it serves different immune response functions. In the bone marrow, lymphoid tissue is responsible for the synthesis of B lymphocytes which fight infections (American Cancer Society, 2013). Therefore, suppressed bone marrow activity leads to increased pathogenic activity in the body. This is the situation involved in immunodeficiency-related Burkitt lymphoma in which immunosuppressive drugs reduce the synthesis of B cells in the bone marrow. In most cases, lymphomas are believed to start in the bone marrow, especially in endemic Burkitt lymphoma which affects the jaw and facial bone.

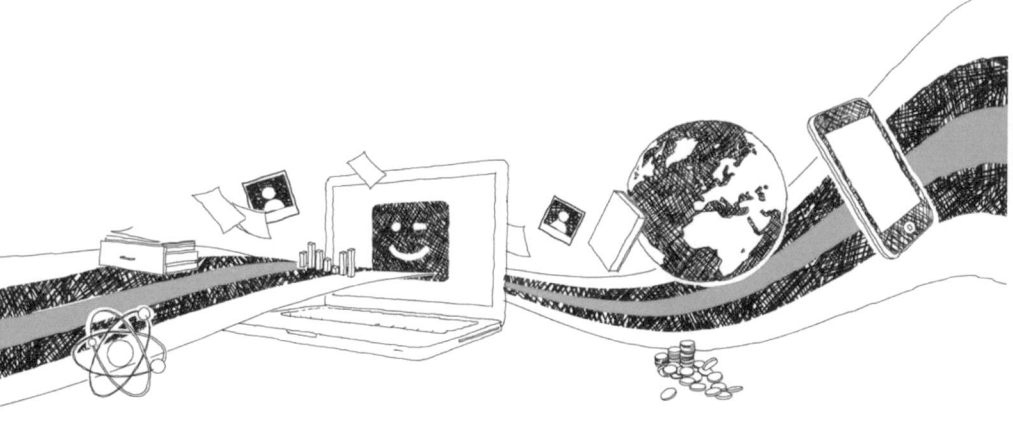
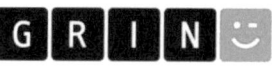

Bibliografische Information der Deutschen Nationalbibliothek:

Die Deutsche Bibliothek verzeichnet diese Publikation in der Deutschen National-
bibliografie; detaillierte bibliografische Daten sind im Internet über http://dnb.d-
nb.de/ abrufbar.

Impressum:

Copyright © 2016 GRIN Verlag, Open Publishing GmbH
Druck und Bindung: Books on Demand GmbH, Norderstedt Germany
ISBN: 978-3-668-24081-0

Dieses Buch bei GRIN:

http://www.grin.com/de/e-book/334252/der-wiener-kongress-und-seine-folgen-
fuer-europa

Bild Europa 1812(Zuletzt besucht am 11.03.2016)

- Wgsebald
  http://www.wgsebald.de/napo/karteu.jpg

Territoriale Neuordnung; Zitat Machtansprüche sind geogr. Ausbreitung
(Zuletzt besucht am 11.03.216)

- LeMO
  https://www.dhm.de/lemo/kapitel/vormaerz-und-revolution/wiener-kongress/neuordnung-europas-181415.html

Personalunion (Zuletzt besucht am 26.02.2016)

- Duden

  http://www.duden.de/rechtschreibung/Personalunion

Deutscher Bund (Zuletzt besucht am 25.03.2016)

- Deutsche-Schutzgebiete
  http://www.deutsche-schutzgebiete.de/deutscher_bund.htm

Heilige Allianz (Zuletzt besucht am 25.03.2016)

- Wissen.de
  http://www.wissen.de/lexikon/heilige-allianz

Deutsch-Französischer Krieg(Zuletzt besucht am 30.03.2016)

- Geschichte-Lexikon.de

  http://www.geschichte-lexikon.de/deutsch-franzoesischer-krieg.php

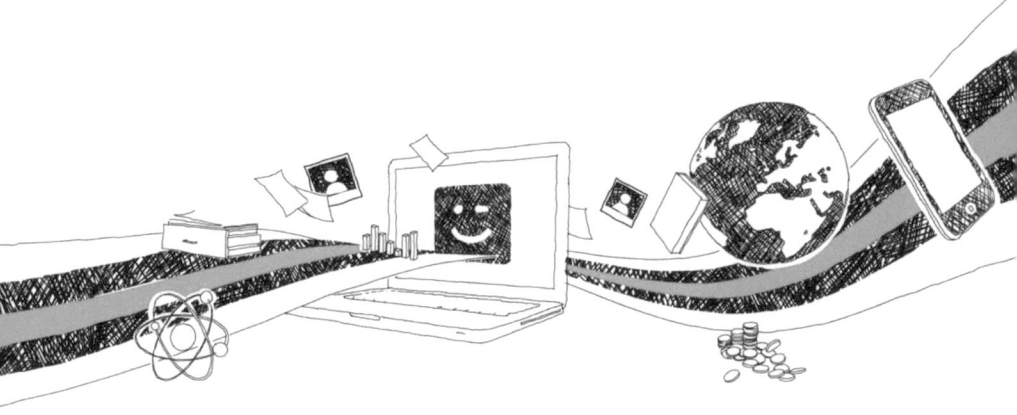
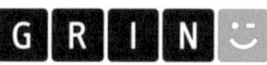

Risk Factors of Burkitt Lymphoma

In theory, all non-Hodgkin's lymphomas share similar risk factors although some may be associated to a given risk factor more or less the same as other lymphomas. Currently, an array of risk factors for Burkitt lymphoma has been identified although the mechanisms behind some risk factors remain unknown. Burkitt lymphoma exhibit similar features to those observed in other forms of cancer although they differ significantly in regard to etiology and risk factors. Some of the risk factors which are believed to increase an individual's chance of developing Burkitt lymphoma include age, gender, immune system deficiency, infections and exposure to certain chemicals. Moreover, lifestyle changes are also associated to the occurrence of non-Hodgkin's lymphoma including Burkitt lymphoma although research studies on the issue provide contradictory evidence.

Age has always been associated with the prevalence of lymphomas. In Burkitt lymphoma, children are the most affected, especially in endemic Burkitt lymphoma which is highly prevalent among children in Africa. However, it is worth noting that the high prevalence rate in African children can be attributed to the severity of malaria in this region. It is reported that, malaria causes the highest disease burden in Sub-Saharan Africa in which children below the age of 5 are affected. In reality, Burkitt lymphoma develops in children who experience malaria episodes because malaria weakens their immunity.

In regard to gender, Burkitt lymphoma occurs more often in boys than girls, primarily in endemic lymphoma cases. Research indicates that, the prevalence of endemic Burkitt lymphoma is twice boys as in girls, especially those aged 4 to 7 years (WebMD, 2013). However, it is worth noting that other forms of Burkitt lymphoma do not show gender as a predisposing risk factor, although research reports reveal a significant correlation between non-Hodgkin's lymphoma and gender in which men are more affected than women (American Cancer Society, 2013).

Exposure to chemicals has been linked to the occurrence of most non-Hodgkin's lymphomas including Burkitt lymphoma. It has been reported that, patients who used chemotherapy drugs for the treatment of other forms of cancer have an increased risk of developing Burkitt lymphoma than those who have never been under cancer treatment chemotherapy. It is also people who were treated for other forms of non-Hodgkin's lymphoma have an increased risk of developing Burkitt lymphoma later in their lives, although it is not certain whether the onset of the disease is caused by the previous condition or its therapy. In addition, patients have been exposed to radiation, especially during radiotherapy treatment have been found to have increased risk of developing Burkitt lymphoma more or less the same as it is the case in other non-Hodgkin's lymphoma (American Cancer Society, 2013).

On the other hand, infections which cause chronic immune system stimulation or weaken the immune system have been found to increase the risk of developing Burkitt lymphoma. As noted earlier, HIV infection plays a pivotal role in the transformation of B lymphocytes into cancerous cells in immunodeficiency-related Burkitt lymphoma (American Cancer Society, 2013). On the other hand, infections which cause constant activation of the immune system are believed to increase the risk of Burkitt lymphoma, more or less the same as in other forms of non-Hodgkin's lymphoma. For instance, *Helicobacter pylori* has been found to increase the risk of lymphomas owing to its ability to cause ulcers in the stomach. This explains the reason as to why mucosa-associated lymphoid tissue lymphoma occurs most in people with *H. pylori* infection. *Campylobacter jejuni* has also been found to increase the risk of developing sporadic Burkitt lymphoma which affects the lower abdomen. Research indicates that *Campylobacter jejuni* infections are responsible for lymphoma prevalence in eastern Mediterranean region in which young adults are the most affected. In addition, hepatitis C viral infection is also believed to cause increased risks of developing non-Hodgkin's lymphoma including Burkitt lymphoma (American Cancer Society, 2013). Moreover, body weight and diet have also been found to play a significant role in increasing the risk of lymphomas, especially in obese people. In addition, dietary regimes with high levels of fat and beef products cause increased risk of lymphoma.

Pathophysiology

The pathophysiology of Burkitt lymphoma encompasses some complexity because there are quite a number of things which have not yet been understood about how these cancers occur. However, there has been some progress in research which has led to the unraveling of some mysteries associated to Burkitt lymphoma and other forms of non-Hodgkin's lymphoma in general. For instance, scientists have identified the mechanism involved in the transformation of normal B-lymphocytes into lymphoma cells and this phenomenon is associated to some changes in an individual's genomic material. It is believed that oncogenes and suppressor genes play a significant role in DNA changes observed in Burkitt lymphoma. In theory, oncogenes are responsible for speeding up cell division for cellular proliferation or organ development. On the other hand, suppressor genes, also known as tumor suppressor genes are responsible for controlling cell death by slowing down cell division. These two processes occur uniformly to ensure efficient growth and development, but fatal consequences occur when imbalances are experienced. In most cases, DNA changes occur during cell division in which the DNA replicates into two replicas before an existing cell divides into two new copies (American Cancer Society, 2013). However, such replication processes are not perfect, so errors occur at times through DNA mutations, which produce abnormal DNA molecules. This implies that some genes on chromosomes are affected. One of the most common DNA mutations involves deletion or duplication of genes.

In theory, Burkitt lymphoma is caused by DNA mutations, which affect the principal genes controlling cell division and cell apoptosis. It is believed that, the transformation of normal B lymphocytes into cancerous lymphomas is caused by two principal mechanisms. First, DNA mutations lead to the stimulation of oncogenes which means they are turned on to promote cell division and proliferation. The second mechanism involves the turning off of the tumor suppressor genes which regulates cell deaths. In most cases, these DNA changes are caused by chromosomal translocations in which some fragments of a chromosome breaks off and attaches on another chromosome causing the impairment of the genes located within the affected chromosome region (American Cancer Society, 2013). As a result, the lymphoid tissue is over stimulated to produce B-lymphocytes when oncogenes are turned on, or old B-lymphocytes experience delayed destruction leading to further DNA changes.

In Burkitt lymphoma, malaria infection, Epstein-Barr virus infection and activation of C-myc oncogene are believed to be responsible for the pathophysiology of the disease although the mechanism involved in the development of most non-Hodgkin's lymphomas has not yet been known.

EBV acts as an etiological agent on Burkitt lymphoma, especially endemic and sporadic Burkitt lymphoma. Endemic Burkitt lymphoma is known to be, predominantly caused by Epstein-Barr virus. Research shows that all patients suffering from endemic Burkitt lymphoma are EBV positive while 20% of patients with sporadic Burkitt lymphoma test positive for EBV. It has been found out that EBV infects B-lymphocytes and enters the germinal center where it causes DNA changes, which lead to excessive B-lymphocyte proliferation (Kanbar, 2016).

On the other hand, malaria infection plays a significant role in the pathogenesis of Burkitt lymphoma, primarily endemic Burkitt lymphoma and immunodeficiency-related Burkitt lymphoma. In theory, malaria infection is believed to influence the immune system responses towards Epstein-Barr virus. It is believed that EBV-specific immune response is inhibited by plasmodium infection by causing abnormal interaction between cellular microRNA (miRNA) and viral RNA. These interactions influence gene expression in the lymphoid cells which in turn interferes with normal translation of RNA into proteins for new B-lymphocytes.

It is also believed that, EBV inhibits the activity of tumor suppressor genes of B-lymphocytes because it produces some proteins which possess anti-apoptotic properties. For instance, EBV-encoded RNAs and EBV nuclear antigen-1 (EBNA-1) inhibit apoptosis process in lymphoid tissues. On the other hand, BCL-2 protein in lymphocytes which acts as anti-apoptotic agent during cell proliferation is inhibited by EBNA-3C AND EBNA-3A produced by Epstein-Barr virus leading to the transformation of normal lymphocytes into cancerous cells (Kanbar, 2016).

Moreover, C-myc oncogene activation in Burkitt lymphoma is believed to be caused by reciprocal gene translocations between chromosome 8 and 14. Chromosome 2 and 22 are also involved in these translocations which cause the activation of C-myc oncogenes. Research shows that, 80% of Burkitt lymphoma is caused by translocation t(8;14) in which C-myc oncogene on chromosome 8 undergoes transposition on chromosome 14 resulting into the activation of C-myc oncogene, which is responsible for tumor proliferation in the lymphoid tissue. On the other hand, translocation t(8;2) and t(8;22) causes gene changes in chromosome 2, primarily on the kappa light chain of the immunoglobulin (Hudson, Link & Weinstein, 2007). Therefore, gene changes in immunoglobulin chains leads to the activation of C-myc oncogenes involved in the transformation of normal lymphocytes into tumor cells.

Activation of C-myc oncogenes leads to the overproduction of C-myc proteins, which influence the expression of p53 gene and DAP-kinase. These two products are involved in cell apoptosis in which they slow down the process of cell division. C-myc proteins are also believed to act as transcription factors during the cell cycle, including differentiation, growth, adhesion and apoptosis. Research indicates that, C-myc gene overexpression leads to the induction of TRAP1, cyclin D2 and HLA-DRB1 genes while PDGFR-alpha production is repressed leading to the formation of lymphomas (Kanbar, 2016).

Physiological Effects of Burkitt Lymphoma Symptoms

In general, Burkitt lymphoma involves the central nervous system and bone marrow. However, there are diverse physiological changes related to the different forms of Burkitt lymphoma. For instance, endemic Burkitt lymphoma cause deformation on the jaw and facial bone in which the orbit is commonly affected leading to the protrusion of the underlying bone (Hoyt, Miller & Frank, 2005). On the other hand, sporadic Burkitt lymphoma presents its manifestations in the abdomen in which abdominal tumors develop, although it involves the bone marrow. In immunodeficiency-related Burkitt lymphoma, nodal formation in the lymphoid system serves as significant manifestations of the disease.

It is believed that abdominal masses are responsible for abdominal distension and pain which is experienced by patients with Burkitt lymphoma. Intestinal perforation and gastrointestinal bleeding, which are accompanied with acute abdomen signs and symptoms are witnessed in Burkitt lymphoma cases. As a result, patients experiences loss of appetite, nausea and vomiting (Kanbar, 2016). Breathlessness and diarrhea are also regarded as some of the most significant symptoms of Burkitt lymphoma.

In the case of endemic Burkitt lymphoma, mandibular masses serve as the principal manifestation of the disease in which 15-20% cases involve the orbit. In most cases, meningeal infiltration, headache, paraplegia and visual impairment serve as some of the most significant manifestations of the disease. It also involves the so-called B systemic symptoms which include fever, fatigue, night sweats and weight loss owing to the impairment of various physiological processes. However, it is worth noting that, Burkitt lymphoma can present itself as painless lymphadenopathy, especially in adults and this complicates its diagnosis (Kanbar, 2016).

Treatment of Burkitt Lymphoma: How Therapies Affect Physiology

Treatment of Burkitt lymphoma involves target therapies, which inhibit the expression of variant genes. Chemotherapy has always been used as the principal therapeutic approach in treating Burkitt lymphoma, in which different drugs has been developed to destroy cancerous cells by enhancing their destruction by the immune system.

On the other hand, monoclonal antibody therapy involves the use of monoclonal antibodies. These monoclonal antibodies designed to recognize cancerous cells and induce an immune response reaction which leads to the destruction of the cells. They also stimulate the immune system to mount cell-mediated immune response against cancerous B cells through the use of macrophages in which monoclonal antibodies stick on the surface of the cancerous B cells for the identification of the variant cells by macrophages (Macmillan Cancer Support, 2013).

Moreover, the treatment of Burkitt lymphoma involves the use of stem cell therapy. In stem cell therapy, stem cells are obtained from a donor and introduced into the lymphoid systems of the patient whereby they differentiate into normal B-lymphocytes to replace malignant cells and restore the normal functioning of the immune system.

Conclusion

Conclusively, Burkitt lymphoma is one of the most prevalent forms of cancer. Its epidemiology exhibits demographic variations in which populations in malaria-endemic regions such as Africa are the most affected. In Africa, endemic Burkitt lymphoma is found, predominantly among children in whom it causes the formation of masses on the jaw and facial bone. It is believed that, endemic Burkitt lymphoma is associated with EBV and malaria infection. Sporadic Burkitt lymphoma, which occurs outside Africa, is also linked to Epstein-Barr virus although the mechanism is not clearly understood. In immunodeficiency-related Burkitt lymphoma, the transformation of normal B-lymphocytes into cancerous cells occurs due to the effect of immunosuppressive drugs used in the treatment of HIV/AIDS or organ transplant.

In general, the pathophysiology of Burkitt lymphoma is attributable to DNA changes in the lymphoid cells in which translocations interfere with gene expression. In most cases, DNA changes lead to the activation of oncogenes or repression of tumor suppressor genes which affect B-cell proliferation and apoptosis, respectively.

References

American Cancer Society (2013). *Non-Hodgkin Lymphoma.* Retrieved from http://www.cancer.org/acs/groups/cid/documents/webcontent/003126-pdf.pdf

Kanbar, A. (2016). *Burkitt Lymphoma and Burkitt-like Lymphoma.* http://emedicine.medscape.com/article/1447602-overview#showall

Hoyt, W., Miller, N., & Walsh, F. (2005). *Walsh and Hoyt's Clinical Neuro-ophthalmology, Volume 2.* New York, NY: Lippincott Williams & Wilkins.

Jaffe, E. (2001). *Pathology and Genetics of Tumors of Hematopoietic and Lymphoid Tissues.* Lyon: IARC.

Hudson, M., Link, M., & Weinstein, H. (2007). *Pediatric Lymphomas.* New York, NY: Springer.

Macmillan Cancer Support (2013). *Burkitt Lymphoma.* Retrieved from http://www.macmillan.org.uk/Cancerinformation/Cancertypes/Lymphomanon-Hodgkin/TypesofNHL/Burkitt.aspx

Lights, V., & Yu, W. (2012). *Burkitt Lymphoma.* Retrieved from http://www.healthline.com/health/burkitts-lymphoma

WebMD (2013). *Burkitt Lymphoma.* Retrieved from http://www.webmd.com/cancer/burkitt-lymphoma-prognosis-diagnosis-treatments>

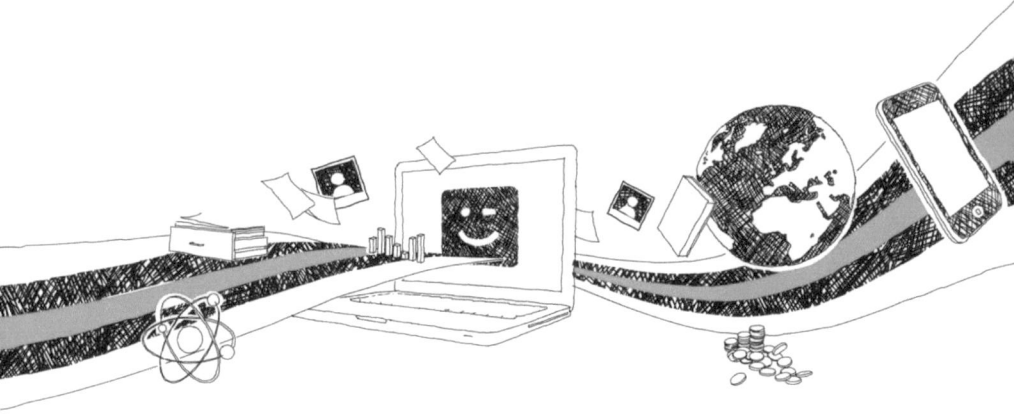
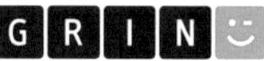